Table of Contents

Challenges and Triumphs: A Parent's Journey with a Child's Multiple Food Allergies

Strategies for Parents: How to Help Your Child with Food Allergies

1. Introduction to Food Allergies in Children

A food allergy is the immune system's response to a food that is either mistakenly seen as a threat or over-reacts to a food protein. In some cases, food allergies can be so severe that just one bite is enough to cause an anaphylactic reaction to a very small percentage of the population. Symptoms from any food allergies can be immediate within minutes to about two hours, but some food allergies can cause a spectrum of delayed reactions that range from behavioral changes to gastritis to severe eczema outbreaks. Even though it can be scary to think about your child having a severe allergic reaction, it is also important to know that the vast majority of reactions are minor. For about 1-2% of the population, their symptoms are severe and life-threatening, and that is what makes them more dangerous.

Food allergies in children have been on the rise in the past decade. It is reported that 8% of children have a food allergy, and approximately 40% of those children have severe enough reactions to warrant time in a hospital emergency room. Although those statistics are alarming, the good news is that many children will grow out of their food allergies, and parents can be a major part of what helps prevent both accidental exposure and anxiety surrounding the food allergy.

2. Understanding Common Food Allergens

Eight major foods or food ingredients cause around 90% of allergic food reactions. These are peanuts, tree nuts, milk, eggs, soy, wheat, fish, and shellfish, which are based on individuals in the United States. Some individuals are allergic to one food, while others may be allergic to two, three, or more. While any food ingredient can provoke an allergy, quite a few foods are responsible for a large majority of problems. In the US, the major food allergens responsible for over 90% of allergic reactions are cow's milk, eggs, fish, peanuts, shellfish (crustaceans and mollusks), soy, tree nuts, and wheat. In the UK, the yellow card schemes require physicians and the public to report single or multi-casual events involving the same allergens. According to the observation log, substances that caused the most repeated symptoms during the last 10 years included: milk-based immune-modifying diets, fruit, tree nut (other than peanut), peanut, sesame, soya (soy), and wheat.

Allergic reactions can occur because of any food, but most commonly, food allergies are initiated by some food items, which are called allergens. A study of 2,211 children with allergies showed that the most prevalent European allergens related to nuts and seeds are peanuts (0.4%–2.2%), tree nuts and seeds (0.2%–1.7%), and sesame (0%–0.88%), followed by fruit (0%–1.1%) and mustard (0%–1.1%). Similarly, in Western countries, common allergens in milk are also prevalent, followed by eggs, soy, grains, fish, and shellfish. Main food allergen components comprised of sequences of amino acids have been discovered, which have been designated as "major allergens" because they occur in a large number of foods and are recognized by IgE in most allergic patients. The most serious and measurable allergens occur in different groups of food items due to the severity of allergic responses. The major food allergens reported as more serious allergens are approximately FB-047 (0.1 to 1.8 mg/mL), FA5 (0.2–3.3 mg/mL), IgE (0.5 mg/mL), and MgCyp (1–3 µg/mL) and rBos d 5 (1.2 µg/mL).

Understand common food allergens

3. Identifying Food Allergy Symptoms in Children

It's helpful to know that food allergy symptoms typically are conjunctive with histamine. For example, if a child is rubbing, picking, or scratching around his mouth after eating foods such as apples, celery, or cherries, it's often due to oral allergy syndrome. Some pediatricians practice sublingual immunotherapy (SLIT), under their guidance, putting the food directly under the tongue which naturally covers the most prevalent allergenic antigens. As the dose under the tongue increases, it's easier to identify if symptoms decrease, stay the same, or increase. Other symptoms of food allergy include coughing, sneezing, runny nose, and watery eyes. These symptoms are generally mistaken for cold-like symptoms, and often are when occurring in a child. Pouring stiff, unforgiving diaries down their throats, children with dairy sensitivities suffer from an instant barking hoarse, phlegmy voice.

It's important for every parent to be able to recognize the myriad of symptoms of a child who might be experiencing an allergic reaction to a food. Symptoms are not limited to itching, swelling, and/or hives. Thankfully, the skin issues tend to be transitory and can fade within a few hours of eating a suspect food. If welting or swelling persists or becomes severe and covers large areas of the body, a pediatrician should be consulted immediately. While a bite from, say, a mosquito can look a lot like an allergic skin reaction, you really don't want to err on the side of taking it more seriously than less. Because every child in the future of the allergic will never have the same symptoms after ingesting a food, symptoms may exhibit days or weeks later after eating the food. At the same time, there are many foods (tree nuts, peanuts, sesame, and soy to name a few) which trigger off multiple symptoms.

4. Diagnosis and Testing for Food Allergies

Allergists are the best place to be diagnosed, as they will guide you in the skin prick tests that usually have high reliability, but they take over an hour to complete. The specific allergens they dip in will be determined by what foods you list for them that you have exposed your child to. Blood tests can also tell you if your body is producing a lot of IgE antibodies, but they might not be accurate in children. This is why allergists favor entering via the skin tests. If medications are being used by your child, they need to be off the medication; there are timelines for how long depending on what medications they are (two weeks to three days is their half-life), so the allergists will give you the timeline for each child. If the allergist gives your child the skin test and they don't react to anything, your child isn't allergic to these foods. If your child does react to something, they can do blood tests and advise you on the next steps.

Diagnosis and testing for food allergies A food allergy diagnosis can be somewhat complicated because allergy tests can have false positives. Since this is the case, only a qualified healthcare provider should enter by themselves or alongside someone who is proficient in food allergies. Contact your child's school nurse if you aren't sure who to talk to. They should have a solid connection with people who can give you good advice, and you want to approach it from a scientific and professional perspective, not an alarmist one.

Pathophysiology of food allergies When your body is trying to fight off the proteins in foods, it will release chemicals like histamines that can cause a variety of symptoms. If the symptoms are mild, it may be due to one food only, mild exposure, or a conditional allergy. A food allergy is not something to be taken lightly, so you should contact your doctor if you believe that you or someone you know may have this issue.

5. Creating a Safe Home Environment for Your Child

Safe and Secure Home Points Great attention must be given to maintaining a safe home environment for the food-allergic child. Here are some practical suggestions to make your home a safe environment for your food-allergic child: - Always have easily accessible two epinephrine autoinjectors. - Designate one individual to administer the epinephrine to the food-allergic child. - Store all required medications together in an accessible area. Someplace that is locked or hard-to-reach is not considered accessible. - You may want to organize your meals so that everyone eats the same basic ingredients. The only addition would be the "allergens" for those that can tolerate them. - Sometimes a family might want to have "allergen-free" areas set up. - You may want to designate a certain pot, pan, and toaster as "allergen-free." - Consider flatware and dishes/containers that are washable in a dishwasher. - Color-coded cutting boards and utensils (to use in your kitchen) for preparing allergen-free and allergic meals could be beneficial. - Allergic plates, cups, and eating utensils could be color-coded. - Draw up a template for a safe kitchen, and attach it to the refrigerator or inside a cabinet. - Always use cutting boards and utensils that are made out of materials that can be thoroughly washed to serve up allergen-free food, i.e. glass, plastic, or artificial stone. - If meats are prepared in advance for someone allergic to a particular meat being cooked, be certain to use a color-coded sheet pan and plastic film to store it in the refrigerator marked with the person's name. - If a microwave is being shared by an allergic child, microwave ovens may need to be cleaned before use by an allergic child. - Use disposable gloves when preparing an allergic child's food in order to cover utensils in-use, without the fear of cross-contamination. - Have robust items like a fire blanket and fire extinguisher on hand and easily accessible. - The kitchen should be cleaned on a regular basis, more often, and more thoroughly for a food-allergic child relative to other persons.

One of the most important strategies for dealing with food allergies is to create a safe environment for your child within your own home. Your home should be a place of safety and relaxation for your child, and even more importantly, a place where you can work and manage effectively any asthmatic and allergic conditions. While you cannot control the food environment outside your home, you can personally guarantee that your home is as allergen-free and safe as possible. This is especially important for young children who eat and play close to the ground where allergens are often found. Be prepared for the work demanded by keeping your home safe for your food-allergic child, but do not wait until you have the problem. It is always best to make any necessary changes at home long before your child comes into the world or before he or she reaches any age when food allergies are diagnosed.

6. Navigating Food Allergies at School and Social Events

It is important to advocate for a supportive environment for your allergic child at school, including an awareness of when food is exchanged, and to be sure that exclusion from food-related activities in alternative foods and celebrations are handled in a manner that does not stigmatize your child. Children with food allergies should be excluded from eating any food provided that may have been contaminated with an allergen. They may always bring in their own safe snack to events in addition to the one supplied by the school. Ask to read the food service or cafeteria menus that are used for the celebration so that your child who packs a lunch can have the equivalent of that day's ingredients.

At school, in daycare, and at other social events, it is essential to communicate your child's food allergies to the staff supervising the event. Arrange a meeting with the appropriate people - the principal, daycare director, or social event planner - to discuss your child's food allergies. Bring your child with you to help him or her understand that the school and family are working together to keep him or her safe. Bring our fact sheet for school personnel with you. Together, develop a Food Allergy Action Plan that includes a few lines about diagnosis, treatment, and the parent's contact information. It also includes a list of foods the child is allergic to, signs of a reaction, what to do if a reaction occurs, and directions for daily management of a food allergy. A standardized plan is also available from your physician to complete.

7. Reading Food Labels and Avoiding Cross-Contamination

8. Meal Planning and Nutritional Considerations

Here are some ideas for alternatives to common allergen-containing foods. Nutritious and safe food choices generally depend on the food allergies of the individual. Even though eggs, milk, and peanuts contain many nutrients, these foods can be substituted for without sacrificing taste and nutrition. Nutrient loss occurs when replacing a food in the diet with an item that does not supply the same vitamins or minerals. For example, a milk-allergic child should drink calcium-fortified rice milk, soy milk, almond milk, and cook with these beverages if the child can tolerate them. Parents are encouraged to experiment with small amounts of a variety of foods and expand their allergic child's diet possibilities. Keep notes to track progress and compare kid-friendly products and recipes to find what works best for your allergic youngster.

To ensure that your child receives the proper nutrients, many parents may find it helpful to consult with a dietitian experienced in food allergies. A dietitian who is familiar with the dietary restrictions of your child's allergens can assist you in developing meal plans or can help provide information about the specific nutritional needs to be aware of when you are shopping or cooking. You can also develop alternative meal plans, shopping lists, or meal ideas that are allergen-free or can be modified easily if necessary. Meal planning will not need to be as strict when your child is eating a broad diet of allergen-free foods, but it may be helpful to start your meal planning by making a list of your child's favorite foods. Then, start planning meals involving those foods and begin to introduce new allergen-free choices to gradually expand your child's diet. By introducing new foods gradually, you can continue to add variety to your child's diet.

9. Building a Support System for Your Family

The support that you get will help to shoulder some of the emotional ramifications of caring for a child who has food allergies. It will offer you another grown-up or two to go to, who can be compassionate and help you problem-solve. It lets you transfer to someone else for a little bit the difficult work of educating and helping your child work out social consequences, and potentially reassure you that your child will have other shoulders to cry on a little later, too. Management will still be focused at home, between you, your child, your pediatric allergist, and your friends and relatives.

No man is an island. Even in contemporary society, in which families often spend a great deal of time apart from their communities, having a solid support system is crucial. A support system is especially important for the family of a child with a food allergy. There are many ways that inactive efforts at building a food-allergy support system with which your family is comfortable can aid food-allergic children. You should include local and long-distance relatives as part of that effort, as well as friends, people at your house of worship or social club, and members of food-allergy online communities who you are particularly fond of. Make sure that everyone who is a likely or occasional caregiver of your child is part of this system. Be honest, open, and informative about your child's food allergies with potential support people.

10. Teaching Your Child to Advocate for Themselves

If someone got onstage to play the piano without any lessons or practicing, it probably would not sound very good. The same goes for teaching food allergy skills to children. As they get older and gain more independence, make sure they can use strategies like washing hands, avoiding handrails, and reading labels. It is a good idea to remind kids of their food allergy rules and how to read labels before sending them off to sleepovers, camp, or a new environment. If your child has multiple caregivers or spends time in different places during the week, it can be helpful to have a reference sheet. Keep a copy for yourself and a copy in your child's backpack or with the caregiver. As they get older, kids can also be trusted with keeping track of a copy of their anaphylaxis action plan. The more comfort they have using it, the more they will remember to use it. Know what your own food allergy rules will be for your child. Consider these possibilities and pray for wisdom. Whether you allow your child to eat something baked alongside (but not baked in) their allergen (like kids' cakes with peanuts baked in the same facility) depends on your comfort level. Your rules may change over time as your child's comfort or self-care abilities change, but stay consistent with your child, and discuss rules with the adults in charge of them.

Teach your child to advocate for themselves: As soon as kids are old enough to understand, teach them the names of their allergens, where they come from, and what other words might be used to describe them. When they can read, have them practice reading labels (you should look first!) to become more aware of where their allergens show up. It is okay to let a child know potential consequences, but it also helps to instill a sense of responsibility. Tell them that they are the ones eating and drinking something, so they need to ask and make an adult aware of questions or concerns they have. When they are old enough, allow them informed and appropriate choices regarding food and social events, with help as needed.

11. Dealing with Emotional and Psychological Impact

To help your child cope, think about how they behave and react in different situations. Talk with them about their feelings and worries; encourage them to talk to you and others about their food allergy; and listen to them. Enlist the help of friends and family who understand and respect the food allergy. Talking about your experiences with a therapist may help you better deal with your emotions. If a therapist is not available in your area, consider speaking to an allergist, who may be able to refer you to a therapist specifically trained in food allergy management. In some cases, families may find support groups such as the Food Allergy Support Group of Minnesota helpful.

People with food allergies and their caregivers live with the threat of reactions every day. This can be an emotional rollercoaster that evokes feelings of anxiety and stress. Children with food allergies may feel different or left out because of the way others treat them or because they can't eat certain foods. They may worry about having an allergic reaction. Of course, this causes a range of emotions for you too. Sometimes, people may not understand the stress and toll that living with food allergy takes. As well, when a child has an allergic reaction, caregivers may experience intense fear, panic, helplessness, and guilt. Parent support organizations can be a great help. Find one that you feel comfortable with and ask other parents for their experiences.

12. Emergency Preparedness and Use of Epinephrine

The Emergency Action Plan for Anaphylaxis associated with the School Zone checklist indicates the standard and point at which epinephrine should be used to treat the allergic reactions. If the individual is experiencing a severe allergic reaction, currently taking antihistamines, experiencing symptoms of severe allergic reaction with difficulty breathing, or currently has mucus in the throat, the following symptoms may indicate the need for the administration of epinephrine. If the child has a second attack after 5-10 minutes without breathing, another dose can be administered while the emergency services are being called. The adrenaline in the epinephrine helps open the airways so that the child can breathe more easily. Additionally, the epinephrine can work to dilate the small vessels in the heart to help the heart work more effectively in combination with the medication's ability to help constrict the small vessels in the body, thereby increasing blood pressure.

Allergic reactions can occur without warning and progress from mild to severe quickly. In this course, it is necessary to present the symptoms of severe allergic reactions and to remember to consult with providers concerning the child's symptoms and medication dosage. It is important to have an emergency action plan and to prepare for possible allergic reactions in advance. Administration of epinephrine is the first and only step listed in all age groups to treat anaphylaxis in the Emergency Care Plan for Anaphylaxis. This is due to the swift and often unpredictable onset of symptoms, as well as the potential for symptoms to worsen in adulthood and with subsequent allergic reactions.

13. Introducing New Foods Safely

Description: Introducing New Foods Safely describes the process of broadening your child's diet by introducing new foods one at a time. Many parents, caregivers, and children with food allergies are eager to broaden a child's diet—especially when the child's diet is limited, the whole family needs to eliminate the allergic food, or there are concerns about nutrient intake. Introduction of new foods may involve discussion of a food challenge, when an allergist gives a child increasing amounts of a food under medical supervision. While this part of the research is still ongoing, there are some small studies which tell us that, for some children, eating small amounts of the allergen on a regular basis can help make allergic reactions less severe.

It may take time to get your child to eat new foods. Here are some ways to do this. Some of these techniques may be supervised or conducted in a clinical setting, such as your allergist's office. This is done for your safety. If investigators think your child is at high risk for a severe food reaction, they will not advise food challenges. Research suggests that eating a small amount of a food that a child is allergic to will help reduce symptoms during allergic reactions—this is called building up tolerance. What some trial researchers are learning is that this can only work if done with the help of a doctor who monitors the child's health.

Introduction

14. Alternative Dining Out Options

Want to give your child more opportunities to eat out and to give yourself and the rest of your family a break from cooking? Try dining at take-out or fast food restaurants. They may have a drive-through instead of dine-in facility, but one of the managers likely has experience in event planning and is assigned a similar position in-store. Most newsletters have space dedicated to featured or new product offerings just for you. Consider gradual exposure through e-mail. Ask the restaurant manager to add your e-mail address to their marketing list. You and your family can visit when free of symptoms, and only if your child is not in an allergy-triggered flare up. Agree on a safe food selection, one that has likely been served without cross-contact with disguised allergens. Start with a clean surface, preferably heated to 'kill' any allergens that may have come into contact before you walk in. Offer a one-time-only offer, perhaps buy six / get six free donuts. Then visit the store on the day of least visitor-activity. Build your experience to the ideal visit - one that is slow in pre-activities like waiting in line to place your order, and faster in the purchase and departure phase. A do-able walk through the 'safe process' of a pleasant trip to a restaurant. Only when you're convinced of the safety based on this online exposure and following the same-can't-go-cheap-rules will you take your child there.

A note to parents.

15. Traveling with a Child with Food Allergies

Your focus when traveling should be on keeping your child's diet as typical as possible. Make sure to pack a wide variety of safe staple foods and plenty of special allergy-free treats appropriate for your child's age. Bring a cooler from home filled with several meals and snacks, but look for some treats at the airport or train station, such as hard candy, fruit roll-ups, gummy worms, lemonade, or soda, that might be appropriate and give you some options on the go. When flying, make all personnel involved in your travel aware of your child's food allergies: the airline when you book your flight; the reservation or ticketing agent with special instructions; and gate agents at check-in or at your departure. Then, educate the flight attendants once they are on board so that they can make the appropriate announcements. Some parents bring a preview copy of the labels they will need in the country to which they are traveling, especially to non-English speaking countries. Make and print multiple copies in advance. If you speak the language, add an additional page of translated common allergens, such as peanuts, and have your child's photo on it. Plan ahead for off-site dining. If you're staying somewhere with a kitchen, cook and eat meals in your residence, or book a reservation. If neither of those is an option, pack safe foods and plan to picnic.

As a parent of a child with food allergies, you have to consider how to feed your child safely in unfamiliar environments, something that requires additional planning, time, equipment, and supplies. However, parents travel with allergic children every day. Here are a few tips to make it easier.

16. Educating Family Members and Caregivers

Make up a second letter that you present to your child's class and their parents to explain the reasons of singling out your child in his/her allergy rules. Should you have any other relatives or a childcare provider, you should make sure that they are very aware of your child's preferences and allergies. They should also be trained in reading ingredient labels, helping your child to become self-sufficient and teach them in label reading as well as the avoidance of problem foods. All children who have demonstrated food intolerance even without physical signs must be checked. Working with these families, the parents and families of children with an intolerance must also hold a discussion about this issue. They should give a food list and educate anyone providing care for them about avoidance tactics and emergency procedures should an allergic response occur.

One of the first steps in keeping your child safe is to educate the family members and care providers of your child. You should talk with your extended family about your child's food allergies and always keep them updated. Many family members may not understand a child's food allergies, so providing them with information or resources can help break down their discomfort. This could be a helpful issue to discuss in the pediatrician's office. You could ask your child's doctor to supply you with a letter or some brochures to give to your child's babysitter, grandparents, or old siblings. This letter or brochure could cover the same ground as the one you give to school.

17. Managing Food Allergies in Adolescents

A 16-year-old girl who was very sensitive to her peanut allergy learned to manage both her risks and those risks she faced from other allergic individuals. Beginning in adolescence, youth spend more time volunteering and seeking part-time job opportunities outside the home. When they do this, they may receive little or no guidance from parents in advance as to what to say and do about their food allergies. Even when parents do give general advice, adolescents may not be ready to recognize the place of food allergy management in their daily lives. While neither approach is best for all teenagers with food allergies, many will benefit from a dual approach. In adolescence, helping youth cope with their food allergies, especially when out in the world, requires parents to use new strategies. Keep talking to your teenagers, especially about daily management of food allergies.

Adolescence is a time of many changes for both youth and parents. During adolescence, peers, rather than parents, increasingly influence the activities and life choices of most youth. Adolescents with food allergies are no exception. Adolescents also generally seek increased independence from their parents in managing their daily activities, such as their food intake and the places they go. Adolescents with food allergies want increased control over the management of and decisions regarding their food intake and the activities they participate in. To be sure, most adolescents with food allergies report regularly avoiding known food allergens; this suggests that they are able to make good choices. However, over 50% report ignoring food allergy warnings at least once. For adolescents, food allergies can still conflict with their goals of fitting in, seeking more independence from their parents, and simply enjoying the pleasure of eating. Like all adolescents, adolescents with food allergies need guidance.

18. Resources and Organizations for Support

There are many organizations that support families dealing with food allergies. Some food allergy groups also provide telephone or email support lines alternatively attend support groups in local communities. Some advocacy organizations can help individuals with a form letter to prevent exposure to allergens during travel. Whether dealing with food allergy, celiac disease, diabetes, or other dietary restrictions, plan a vacation that will accommodate your needs, such as a cruise or resort. Support groups are a good source for information on safe places to dine and find safe food products. Many mental health or counseling professionals facilitate support groups. Additionally, search for local or regional online food allergy resources. Parents or organizations that have experience with food allergies may share information regarding local resources, dining establishments, grocery stores, and information about individuals who prepare allergen-safe meals.

Food allergies require consistent and ongoing attention to avoid exposure to allergens, which is hard for children to do on their own. Parents often express concerns about leaving their children in the care of others or sending them to school because of their food allergies. Though many caregivers are understanding and very supportive of food allergies, insufficient knowledge and understanding about food allergies can lead to unintentional exposure. Therefore, part of keeping food-allergic children safe is finding support for yourself as a parent. These resources provide families with care, community, and great advice!

19. Research and Developments in Food Allergy Management

Treatment can be groundbreaking if approved by the FDA to begin the process of actively managing your child's allergies. Thanks to the groundbreaking research conducted in the areas of food allergy research and treatment in the last 10 to 20 years, physicians, experts, researchers, and allergists have a large, diverse body of knowledge with which they can draw on when dealing with food allergies. Researchers and scientists will leverage this knowledge to continue treatments and other forms of research to enable them to best assist individuals who are living with food allergies on a daily basis. In some cases, different products that were researched or in the process of getting FDA approval come to market. These are very under-explored areas for food allergies, including further research into the causes of food allergies, advances that can significantly reduce the chance for kid "with permission" forms, which are incredibly traumatic for parents - life or death situations. Some of the latest studies suggest protection or decreased likelihood of exposure or a child's sensitivity to that ingredient. They actively expose children in a monitored environment to the ingredient over time to see whether that buildup of exposure can lead to allergic histamines or a reaction.

Research and developments in food allergy management provide insights into the latest advancements in food allergy research and management, including new treatments and different options that are currently in the research pipeline.

20. Frequently Asked Questions (FAQs)

3. Why do so many foods cause allergies? No one knows for sure, because the mechanism of food allergies (the allergic antibody IgE binding to large pieces of ingested food which appear in the blood and causes allergic reactions) is unusual. This antibody, and the factors that control the production of IgE antibody, are hereditable.

2. Did I do something to cause my child's food allergies? Highly unlikely. Symptoms of food allergy might worsen slightly if eaten by a breastfeeding mother or formula-drinking infant, which might further irritate the gastrointestinal tract, if not totally healed. Pregnant women avoid foods known to cause allergic reactions and symptoms in the pregnant woman, if not the newborn baby, during the breastfeeding period. But, the cause of food allergic reactions appears to be the result of many complex interactions between heredity and environment.

1. How do I find out what my child is allergic to and is it necessary to eliminate many foods? The most reliable, but not the only, method is through allergy skin testing and blood allergy testing ordered by a doctor. Eliminating only those foods which your child is found to be allergic to can be helpful. It is not necessary to eliminate very many foods simply because food allergies are suspected or because there is the common impression that "my child must be allergic to something in their diet because their rash does not improve."

Frequently Asked Questions

Challenges and Triumphs: A Parent's Journey with a Child's Multiple Food Allergies

1. Introduction

I remember the first time my husband and I were told our son had a food allergy. As new parents, we were ripe for worry and uncertain. We asked so many questions. The allergist said, "Don't worry, only a small percentage of people have a reaction." As we continued to adjust to the demands of managing food allergies, we had many successes and even more failures and reactions. We are our children's advocates, and we know that by spreading awareness, we are, in the end, helping him. It's been a rollercoaster, but one that we would both flip and ride again. When we look back at everything that Christian has gone through, we can't help but feel pleased and proud of how far he has come. In this story of our son and his allergies, we have been privy to the world of food, parenting, and simply how life unfolds when it doesn't meet our expectations.

The journey wasn't something I expected. It wasn't on my radar that my child would have multiple food allergies. At 14 months old, my son was diagnosed with over 20 food allergies, including dairy, eggs, wheat, peanuts, and tree nuts. Over time, he has outgrown most of his allergies and now only has four (milk, eggs, soy, and peanuts). About three years ago, he was also diagnosed with Eosinophilic Esophagitis, an allergic inflammatory condition of the esophagus. It's been a tough journey with many ups and downs; each day was a new challenge. Although he has overcome so much, in a way, his journey has only just begun. What happens when the lights turn on? Surprises can still come around the corner, and I know we must still be prepared for any change or challenge that comes his way.

1.1. Overview of the Topic

In a culture with strong family, friend, and community bonds, 'feeding' is central to celebrating within a variety of cultures. Because of this, enjoying holiday gatherings, birthday parties and baby showers, or even dining out together presents unique concerns for most food-allergic families. However, the triumphs that are won with every small victory are usually all the more sweet to those families who contend with managing multiple food allergies. Identifying effective strategies and gathering them together, empowering themselves and those children in their care, promote courage, teach compassion, and bring wisdom and strength to the entire family. Deciding to bring a child into their homes truly rejuvenates us and reminds us of the possibilities in life. These decisions as parents, no matter our individual circumstances or responsibilities, make us stronger and braver than we ever thought we could be.

Multiple food allergies can be an isolating thing for a parent as well as a child. Allergies come in all shapes and sizes, and no two families will have the same experience. While it's easy to focus on the negative, it is important to also pay attention to all the positive aspects of being the parent of a child with (or children with) multiple food allergies. Whether it is new milestones being met or new lessons learned, raising children with multiple food allergies yields many highs as well as many lows.

2. Understanding Multiple Food Allergies

Many people will take this long, albeit insufficient, list of offending foods and begin the arduous process of trying to eat them. When we started treating and talking about this condition twenty years ago, these were the only options available for the parents and children confronting multiple food allergies. To say there have been triumphs in that time period would be a gross understatement. For instance, the FDA approved a desensitization therapy for peanuts and began a rolling review of a desensitization therapy for egg. Researchers discovered the microbiota of a healthy infant has a distinct trajectory from a child with multiple food allergies and children with peanut allergy are reportedly sensitized to the peanut 2s Albumin, not the Ara h 1. In other words, just as Mark Twain commented about how everyone talks about the weather but no one does anything about it, both medical research and treatment have taken multiple food allergies much more seriously now that they have a name and are seen all over the world.

Multiple food allergies occur when a person's body has an adverse, often immune-based, reaction to several types of food. The human race does not entirely understand this process. Common food allergens that can affect an individual suffering from multiple food allergies are cow's milk, gluten, eggs, shellfish, nuts, and soy. The symptoms of multiple food allergies can range from digestive complaints, hives, or itching to anaphylactic shock. Doctors diagnose through blood tests and skin tests to check for IgE-mediated allergies. A doctor will also rule out celiac disease before determining if a patient has true food allergies, which can be diagnosed through an elimination diet or through a blood test that checks for food-specific IgG antibodies.

2.1. Common Food Allergens

Although many food allergens are defined for adults, especially in certain ethnic groups, they are especially pertinent for children. This essay focuses on common foods that can lead to allergic reactions when ingested. The focus is particularly on foods of relevance to parents dealing with multiple food allergies in children. Results are discussed in relation to parents' accounts of their child's multiple food allergies. In this study, dairy products include cow's milk, cheese, milk, yogurt, and eggs. Fish includes tuna, salmon, and shellfish. Shellfish includes crab, lobster, and shrimp. Tree nuts include almonds, cashews, and peanuts. Soy is a type of bean, and peas are legumes; both are not allergenic for anaphylaxis.

The most common foods are eggs, fish, milk, peanuts, shellfish, soy, tree nuts, and wheat. The most common foods often differ; they are called typical foods for a region. In the U.S., the most common foods leading to food allergies are cow's milk, peanuts, eggs used in a variety of foods, fish (such as shellfish, but not usually crustaceans), soy, tree nuts, and wheat. Some allergies can be so severe that even the tiniest bit of the food can cause a serious reaction. Because of their widespread presence, these allergens must be labeled in packaged foods (see Section 1.5). Some people avoid trigger foods they have never even tried because of concern about potential severe reactions. Food allergens vary depending to some extent on the individual reactions of the person and common foods in the region.

2.2. Symptoms and Diagnosis

After developing food allergy symptoms, the only way to check your child's allergies is to undergo a food allergy test by a healthcare provider. Tests that are often used to track food allergies in infants include skin-prick tests, blood tests, the oral food test, and what is sometimes called a food challenge. Because these tests are interpreted by trained doctors, seek an evaluation if you are concerned that you or your child has a food allergy. The oral food test or "food challenge" is the only way to diagnose an allergy conclusively. Under the control of a doctor, the patient returns to a normal diet. As soon as the patient's body has adjusted to the medication, the tests yield the most reliable results. In fact, a "planned" reaction as a symptom of the allergy rather than an unplanned one probably gives the food challenge's most accurate results. These symptoms are then carefully watched and treated. The patient's immune response to foods is usually one of the diagnostic tests. Skin tests and blood tests are both popular options to check. Skin tests are a type of direct test in which drops of actual purified proteins of specific foods are put on the person's forearm or back.

Food allergy is more common than one would expect and begins with a variety of symptoms. Skin is where allergies commonly make their first appearance. Full-body rashes of many types, from hives to eczema to overly dry skin, can appear in allergic children. Other skin symptoms can include excessively red cheeks or rashes that appear soon after consuming certain foods. Gastrointestinal symptoms can also be a clue that an allergy is affecting an infant. Colic, vomiting, and diarrhea are gastrointestinal symptoms and undiagnosed food allergies in young children, but they can also occur for other reasons. Swelling in the throat and trouble breathing may occur in a serious allergic reaction called anaphylaxis.

3. Impact on Daily Life

Parents not only help their child manage the impact the allergies have on them, but they also have to deal with how those effects will spill over to other aspects of life, including social and emotional ones. Socially speaking, not all extended families or friends understand the implications food allergies may have on a parent, especially when these individuals have a limited knowledge or experience with potentially life-threatening allergies. A child is less likely to be invited to a birthday party, a play date, or an overnight get-together. They sense the potential implications of consuming an unknown allergen when anxiety levels escalate upon being asked if a certain food is safe. A parent feels the guilt of asking and sadness upon the realization that a child may never attend such an event, missing seeing a child's happy face. Different settings and environments with the education and management of a multiplicity of food allergies make different impressions on a child.

When a child is diagnosed with more than one food allergy, the daily routine of this family often shifts drastically. Suddenly, emphasis is placed on what is in each item at the local grocery store, rather than what is forgotten on the list at home. There are challenges involved in finding the best allergen-safe substitute for favorite foods. The daily meal planning process transforms unintended chefs into professional background checkers. Continual phone calls, unanswered emails, and inconveniently placed 800 numbers turn hope into triumph when a representative assists in identifying a safe allergen product or when wireless internet access is available to verify ingredients.

3.1. Meal Planning and Preparation

Trying to get her to eat "weird" foods is not an option; I must make replacements for her parts of our meal if she will not eat them. Preparing for her meals is challenging because she will not eat so many foods and textures, she gets sick of foods so easily, we are on a tight budget and must purchase items that are expensive and find places to purchase them, and we must account for all of the supplements and extra vitamins she must take due to her diet and malabsorption of vital nutrients. I must take the time to plan all of our meals, shopping trips, and think in advance for "what ifs" and possible food purchases I may need to make and where. Every day is a balance of trying to keep her food interesting and new and not too overwhelming while not boring or disgusting.

For the past two years, my husband and I have learned to cope with our daughter's multiple food allergies. Meal planning and preparation are the two most challenging components of dealing with her allergies, not only because she has multiple allergens to which she reacts, but also because she will only eat certain foods to begin with. Prior to her allergies, she was a very picky eater and not a good eater, but now she is a healthy dose of picky with an ample appetite. Complicating our meal preparation is the fact that we are a family of five and must take care of everyone's unique palate while coping with the foods we must exclude due to Liesl's allergies. Prior to and during meal preparation, we must consult with Liesl so she can request the brand or variety of food she would like. I must consult with her to ensure that I am making a dish that she will even eat. I must prepare a deviant plan for her.

3.2. Social and Emotional Challenges

Eating out was the most challenging for CJLER families, largely a result of menu substitutions and the anxiety associated with potentially life-threatening food. For some, the fear of new reactions made the prospect of eating at a public place too risky. In time, some parents and their children would "get hives in their mouth or swelling when eating out," which led to anxiety. Parents described feeling that they "were always on edge when eating in a restaurant." When dining out, some parents would participate in extensive preparation, such as calling ahead of time to ask detailed questions about ingredients and to ensure that the restaurant could serve safe food or bring their own food to the restaurant. All of this anxiety and effort resulted in many families opting for take-out instead of dining in. Overall stress and anxiety were commonly reported with this struggle.

Socially, the management of milk and egg allergies made feeding and child care, and eating out a challenge. Upon diagnosis, some families reported feeling as though they "were in a completely different world from other parents." Participants talked about the difficulty navigating common social situations (like playdates or birthday parties) and adjusting to the social exclusion associated with partaking in the food offered at these events. Often, to handle birthdays or gatherings, parents would feed their child prior to an event to allow their child to participate without eating. In other cases, they would bring safe food for their child or ask the hosting parent of the event to provide alternative snacks. They could no longer "grab breakfast before school" or "pop into a restaurant with friends" because of their child's allergies. Children were additionally described as "excluded and left out" at birthday parties or school events where allergens were being served. Because of these barriers, families often felt isolated and had to organize their own social events to accommodate their child's needs.

4. Navigating the Healthcare System

There are many food allergies, and they can always change. On top of that, foods are not the only things that we can be allergic to. In addition, common food allergy symptoms look a lot like common illnesses. Learn the signs and symptoms of a reaction. The allergist might do some medical tests that other kids do not have. It might hurt a little bit, but it's very important. The allergist needs to do these tests to find out what your child is allergic to so that he can make a plan. The tests also help the allergist watch out for any future problems. Some blood tests check to see if there is any allergy antibody in the blood. There are also "scratch tests." This test puts a little bit of allergen in the dead cells in the top layer of your child's skin. It will feel like a "scratch," and then you're done. The doctor might give your child some special medicine called "medicine challenge." This medicine checks to see if your child is allergic to a certain food. It is very safe!

Navigating the healthcare system. Allergists are good for helping to identify the allergens that are causing your child's symptoms, diagnose food allergies, give treatment plans, prescribe medicines, and help educate you on foods to keep your child away from. If you can, try to find a doctor who specializes in allergies with a focus on children. Just like with every other type of medicine, there are a lot of things to know. Don't worry, you don't need to be a pharmacist to help your child feel better. Be prepared to

see one or many doctors. Your child's food allergies will
cause problems with more than just his tummy.

4.1. Allergists and Specialists

Food Allergies are on the rise, with asthma and atopic dermatitis. In fact, recent studies have demonstrated an alarming increase in the prevalence of asthma, with a 75% increase in asthma rates over 20 years. There is a family-based component to these allergies, and they are much more common in folks born to those allergic parents. Atopic immunoglobulins are released into your blood and the allergic mast cells bind to these antibodies. Inside is a tracheal tube, and on the other side of that is another mast cell filled with chemicals ready to secrete if there is a subsequent allergic reaction to what you have eaten, inhaled or injected. There are many types of allergies, and some of these include food, venom (bee and wasp stings), environmental allergies, including trees, pollens, grasses, dust mites, molds, cats, dogs, horse, rodents, and cockroaches in addition to medications having an associated allegetic pneumonia and fully systemic allergic response as well.

Because Sam's food allergies were so severe, his pediatrician referred us to a pediatric allergist. Specialists such as allergists can be an invaluable resource for parents. We have found them to be the leading experts in learning each of Sam's allergies. An allergist is a medical doctor who is an expert in the diagnosis and treatment of as. Allergists have several additional years of specialized training in the field of allergy and immunology to give them the expertise to know what underlying mechanisms cause these often debilitating symptoms. Not all allergic symptoms are due to allergy, which is why it is important to seek guidance from an allergist when symptoms of allergies are present.

4.2. Medical Tests and Treatments

Once diagnosed, patients are referred for a food allergy education session, they see a dietician or nutritionist, and are followed by a clinical immunology and allergy specialist. A private allergist accepted into a research project may collaborate with an allergist at an academic hospital and attempt food challenges based on outgrowing IG/EG and the introduction of oral food sips in the hospital's day admissions area. A largely private system with support programs in Calgary, Edmonton, and Ontario, allergy sufferers pay significant costs when drugs and devices are not covered, and private insurers refuse coverage. When publicly funded, allergists and pediatric specialists collaborate and work with a dietitian through a provincial health authority. A pemolizumab (Fasenra) treatment is available every 4 weeks as an infusapenia with 38 pre-medications and Fasenra with 5 pre-medications as an autoinjector pen every 8 weeks. Anapen and Emerade are not currently available, and the EpiPen Jr short-juvenile adrenaline autoinjector (E-PIP) is used in children weighing 15-30 kg.

To have a multiple food allergy, particularly to multiple foods that can cause anaphylaxis, drives frequent interaction with various healthcare providers. The diagnosis starts with food and symptom history and a review of test results. Physicians order food-specific IgE skin prick or blood tests, or an oral food challenge, the latter considered the gold standard. Secondary testing may include additional blood tests such as the basophil activation test or specific IgE component testing. If a patient has the appropriate history or results, the referring doctor can order an Epipen and have the patient initiate the registration process with MedicAlert.

5. Educating Family and Friends

It is an art - to educate the family about the allergies. My in-laws were with us in Austin, but when they returned to Pakistan, they really tried to provide our eating regimen for our 3 ½-year-old daughter and allergic son. It got so bad, however, that I feared they might not truly appreciate the entire situation. My fear was tugged on every time they professed the belief that "a little bit won't hurt" when my father-in-law attempted to feed my 7-year-old son even a trace of a peanut. I spoke with my husband, but there was no feasible solution. Our son was three back then; now, at age seven, we are contemplating challenging the nut allergy. My mother-in-law has a very hard time distinguishing herself from others in the loss of flavor-enhancing and thickening ingredients. I can understand this lack of understanding concerning the degree of cross-contamination and why a lipstick covered in peanut oil could never touch my child's skin.

With the physical and emotional pain that food allergies bring, one might expect that circumstances could not get worse. However, when your child has a 'life-sustaining diet' made up of a dozen or two dozen ingredients and several others that cause atopic reactions as well, the entire world is forever changed, and innocuous everyday events become laden with larger-than-life stressors. From the outset, a great deal of energy has been spent maintaining the safety of our home - we checked every food that we owned and made phone calls to all the companies we used. Upon the arrival of foodstuff into our home, we checked the ingredient labels again and again. Reading labels is no mere matter either; before we learned all of the hidden words, we called the producers to make sure that no 'natural flavors' or 'spices' were really there. When the teacher sends candy home with my allergic children, I may have to preside over an entire lesson with the entire class, instructing them on the underlying construct that even candy may constitute a potential threat to my child. Additionally, often I end up giving away the candy at the outset of the class to protect my son.

5.1. Creating Allergy-Safe Environments

Indeed, it is evidence to me, at least, that our trusted minders were never more than their word and ensured that at all times, compost toilet paper was acceptable and ensured. Not one of our friends ever turned their backs on us, with huffy heads decorated in frustration at the efforts they had to make to satisfy our requests for almond-free chocolate. None of our children's invited friends ever grumbled or baulked at requests to wash hands, and some even took it upon themselves to scrutinize labels more closely and put danger-foods out of Àine's reach with enough skill to start a food arranging business. While it is natural, I suppose, during such a distressing and grief-ridden time as the one that families experience when faced with a childhood food allergy, for goodwill to be precious, if these few words help to reassure even one new family that some of the darkness can be diluted and much fun enjoyed, we have made a small enough contribution.

Environments safe and supportive to those with life-threatening allergies are as much a testament to courage as they are a show of strength and determination. From the time Àine was old enough to attend nursery sittings, child-minders, play schools, and hosts alike had to be made acutely aware of her restrictions and necessary allergen-induced avoidance. All the meetings, phone calls, and written expressions of our concerns paid off, however. Not one of the most important people who would become active in Àine's weekly routine was anything but keen to understand, cooperate, and quietly diligent when the time came to put in place avoidance measures. As a stated first choice in care arrangements, I would suggest that no one who is not prepared to rise to this challenge would have been worthy of looking after our delicate charge.

6. Advocacy and Support

It has been breathtaking to watch people put food allergy legislation in place, advocate during hearings, and voice our concern about what is happening in an Anaphylaxis Community. I have been able to lend my own voice and tell my own story in this past year, raising over $16,000 that goes directly to the PuGLIFE Foundation. To do this we have teamed up with Nonallergicindividual.org and are using a new program they have established called "Serve it up: Teens 15 & up for a cause." The kids partake in tournaments and food drop-offs to local emergency rooms, prescribing offices, and schools. They also help the community in different ways like buying animals for third-world countries, donating Christmas trees, signing up bone marrow donors, and many other opportunities. The Give Back Games Nashville trendsetter was Marqui. To learn more about this program and how we can help, please go to nonallergicindividual.org and click on "Serve it up again!" You can also go to Facebook and check out our page "Give Back Games Nashville".

The stress and anxiety begin to alleviate when you meet people who share your day-to-day reality. Consequently, the journey has been greatly influenced by my participation in multiple Facebook support groups. I never fully appreciated the value of support groups in times of crisis until I experienced the solidarity and care offered by complete strangers. It is also incredible how quickly people are willing to provide advice, celebrate your triumphs, commiserate with your struggles, share recipes, and help you brainstorm ideas. It can sometimes be easy to feel isolated dealing with more challenges than the average person. Additionally, advocating for food allergies is another way to drastically influence your perception of managing a life with food allergies.

6.1. Joining Support Groups

I turned to other blogs, websites, and forums where people gathered to talk about living with or caring for those with food allergies. I found a local non-profit group which puts on a series of programs and support group meetings. This group was a godsend in those early days. I met a physical therapist who had a child with multiple food allergies, the leader of the San Francisco area parent support group called POFAK — Parents of Food Allergic Kid(s), and countless others to whom our story resonated. The group met a few times a year and it was always at those meetings that I learned a lot about living with and parenting a food allergic child. It was at those meetings that I made friends with whom I would walk the road ahead.

The need for a supportive community comes up again and again when discussing managing the tricky logistics of having a child with multiple food allergies. It is a lonely, isolating world that one must get used to when the grocery store becomes off-limits for anything besides personal hygiene items and aluminum foil. My advice for fellow parents and families managing this life is to find your people. Join support groups, in-person or online, social media or house meetings, to meet and talk about the trials and tribulations of parenting a child with food allergies. The mothers (and a few fathers) that I have met since my son's diagnosis have made a world of difference in my life. They sympathize, empathize, and offer practical advice.

6.2. Raising Awareness

Pre-Natal Class: Before I even had Ellie, we had to attend a prenatal class put on by our local health unit. It is also offered specifically to parents of babies with food allergies as a way to prepare us for motherhood (pros and cons, introducing solid food). I was a bit concerned by the outdated PoFA recommendations in the presentation in 2007 and was happy to be asked to revamp the PowerPoint. After contesting a few of the ideas, I was told that they start with a blank slate and don't include many of the current, controversial management approaches as they want to prevent conflict, etc. Additionally, the leader of the prenatal program was told that she is there to teach nutrition, so she had great difficulty understanding and teaching the social aspects of living with food allergies.

Support Group: I co-founded a support group for all folks with allergies and sensitivities. Our numbers include people with environmental sensitivities, food allergies, celiac disease, and those with eosinophilic disorders. The weather has turned nicer, so we will hold our first picnic next month. We have been holding regular meetings and have had good attendance. I wrote an article with a good friend and support group co-founder, which should be published in the paper on our picnic day. We were lucky to find a good editor.

Local Media: There have been a couple of articles written in the local newspaper about my daughter and me and our food allergy journey. There have also been a couple of interviews done about our Food Allergy Support Group in the developer community of the magazine.

Second, I started a private Facebook group for parents of kids with food allergies. We have about 26 members, and we share stories, successes, and challenges. It is great to be able to connect.

Facebook: I have a few private groups on Facebook. First, a small group of us food allergy parents at the local school began meeting and talking about sharing our experiences with the broader school community - children, teachers, and parents. One mom in the group was a teacher and thought this would also be a great professional development opportunity for her colleagues. To facilitate this, we thought we could provide our thoughts anonymously. I created a Facebook group called "Anonymous Questions on Severe Allergies in School." We are hoping all of the questions that are posed will also be used to help inform our allergy education presentation we will be giving to approximately 300 middle school kids.

A big part of my journey as a food allergy mom has been to raise awareness about food allergies. Here are some of the ways I have worked to do this.

7. The Role of Schools and Childcare Centers

Do you know what anaphylaxis is? How to recognize it? What to do in response? Chances are high that you do. If your child attends a school, before and after-school program, or daycare, it's quite likely that you have been given a care plan and a 10-minute education by the staff should your kiddo present with anaphylaxis. Children who present at school in anaphylaxis and carry an EpiPen typically have an Allergy Action Plan. In my daughter's preschool years, she had a plan in both Middletown, NJ, Long Island, and Brooklyn, NY. Each action plan accompanied an EpiPen that had a current prescription from a registered allergist, my most recent pediatrician, and then, a Children's Allergy Specialist. Every daycare and community action training provided information on the use of an EpiPen. Everyone talked about using filler foods for birthdays and events, that we have many food allergies, 10, 15, who's counting. These centers were deeply involved in accommodating food allergies. This month is extensive, but keep in mind, I have been dealing with it for a number of years.

Epinephrine - another word to add to my spellcheck list. I've never needed to give anyone epinephrine. I am not an expert in the use of an EpiPen, but I have prepared EpiPens multiple times. Apart from a child care setting, I've also made peanut butter and jelly sandwiches in the middle of a meditative play therapy session for a child I will be working with next week who can only eat this "my safe food." I sigh and laugh at the pure irony of such a statement. A child whose main food source is a staple in my 4-year-old daughter's diet, one of the very few things that I give her for lunches and snacks that invariably makes it back home.

7.1. Developing Allergy Action Plans

The best way to deal with anaphylaxis is through a teamwork approach involving teachers and allergic reaction management. In fact, it was shown that allergists agree that primary schools and kindergartens should always engage parents in the knowledge and management of food allergy, and that teachers, chefs, and all school staff should be informed about anaphylaxis and be prepared to act. In this study, nutritional knowledge of foods and allergens was good, as children suspected of an allergy were temporarily fed during their visits. However, this prescription allowed the children to continue eating allergenic foods at all other "non-programmed" times, even though epinephrine was prescribed by the parents in the event of a serious reaction. This study emphasizes the need for careful support for a child with food allergy before the first day of school. Nutrition education or anaphylaxis will be focused on "accidentally eating forbidden food" in future actions.

Comprehensive allergy action plans use the combined knowledge, skills, and expertise of food allergy management professionals, pediatric allergists, nurses, dietitians, and parents. It is equally important that schools and early childhood settings are aware of the challenges and importance of managing multiple food allergies within their environment, and all are involved in the ongoing reassessment of the allergy management plan. This will enable parents to have confidence that the school environment is regularly reviewed and provides the highest level of protection and support services for their child. Food Allergy & Anaphylaxis Australia encourages and actively works with schools and early childhood settings to be committed to providing allergy and anaphylaxis education and management training. The childcare center is a "nut-free" center, and the focus of future actions on nutrition education or anaphylaxis will be "accidentally eating forbidden food". Measures to prevent the future occurrence of a similar event are presented in an algorithm for the outpatient department. These measures include close cooperation between pediatric outpatient physicians and allergy experts, repeated health education for both children and adults emphasizing the importance of severely allergic food in the child's diet, developing and signing medical letters for schools, helping repercussions of the parents' discussions with each other, and investigation of anaphylaxis with a specialist at the time of referral. I also encourage increased networking between pediatricians and allergists to ensure joint action in clinical practice.

8. Nutrition and Alternative Food Options

We also have to consider alternative food options. For example, a child without a dairy allergy is allergic to almonds. It's almost common sense to suggest the parent choose an almond-based product over dairy. For us, it's not that simple. What if the child is allergic to almonds as well? The parent then may choose, say, hemp or oat milk. Whatever option the parent chooses, it's extremely time-consuming and potentially difficult. We read labels and ingredients for everything we buy – but, as we've learned, we must also do the same for every product we consume at any restaurant. We spend hours at the grocery store, and what's more, the alternative options we have for Xander are not always the best nutritious options or may contain other allergens. In rare cases, even the alternatives we will buy for him specifically are contaminated with allergens.

Another challenge my husband and I have tried to get our minds around is the nutrition for Xander as he grows. A typical child's diet doesn't always contain all the essential vitamins, minerals, and nutrients necessary for a growing child. A child with a limited diet due to multiple food allergies can exacerbate this problem. My husband and I take the responsibility of Xander's diet very seriously and are fortunate to have access to a nutritionist we see on a yearly basis. It is difficult but certainly can be done.

8.1. Reading Labels and Ingredients

Allergen-Free The labels are both needed in nutrition management as one is for individuals having to avoid sesame seeds, while the other product is of high concern for those who cannot eat sweet potatoes/eggplant to manage a child's multiple food allergies. Considering fruit, most packaged items will contain citric acid as a preservative adding to the item's flavor profile. The skin of a fruit can sometimes have a reaction if allergic to either the fruit or within the other allergens above. However, as the fruit sits open to air for a period of time, it can become metallic tasting which the child may not like. From being a chemist that will slightly taste (neutral charge) salt when added to a cup of coffee with stirring, be careful with either the juice, flavor extracts as it is like adding salt to a recipe where you get the sweetness taste hit. Formulation works really well. All of this leads to reading the ingredients for allergies to be comfortable to consume.

Recipes are an inspiration where they can accommodate the individual. Additionally, seeking professional guidance to helping with dietary planning and understanding food allergies is very important for the best nutrition and nutritional adequacy.

To ensure the gluten-free or allergen-free status of a food, the label is the first item to review since this is where food manufacturers must note any declared allergens. Throughout Canada and the United States, the common allergens that must be declared are: peanuts, tree nuts (almonds, Brazil nuts, cashews, hazelnuts, macadamia nuts, pecans, pine nuts, pistachios, and walnuts), milk, eggs, fish, crustacean shellfish, soy, and wheat. With peel-back or package transparency, many whole fruits and vegetables will not have an ingredients list, rather just the ingredient that is within the package itself. Also, it is important to recognize that we all have the same ingredient list on a product. It isn't derived this way for the "allergen community" and that for us it pertains to all of what is to be consumed of a product. If we see that the first ingredient is what we are avoiding, then the consumer should move onto the next product. Let's look at a couple of labels to see, all are whole fruits and vegetables.

9. Traveling with Food Allergies

While researching if a trip can work for you/your child, pay attention to all meal times. If meal times are not within your control, plan to have an easily prepared meal available. For example, if an early morning flight is your only option but your child's mood and health are directly related to having breakfast, a safe meal must be offered. If the symptoms of delayed symptoms from a delayed airplane or being stuck in a tube of germs will be severe for your child, that also would mean adjusting your plans for the trip. You can visit the food allergy menus sites; a quick search for allergy-friendly foods in the area will yield helpful results. Plan your vacation with a kitchen. By always staying places that have a kitchen, you can prepare meals that you know are safe for your children, and yourself, to eat. Since the greatest variety of safe, truly healthy foods can always be prepared from scratch, the kitchen in your accommodations grows in importance here.

Plan ahead. No matter where you are going or how you are getting there, whenever you are planning a trip, consider how you will handle food for your child with food allergies, especially if he is young and you face more restrictions of always needing to carry all of their food with you. The method of travel will help guide you in planning.

9.1. Preparing for Trips

- Preparing for trips: Where are you going and what are you doing? - Lodging - Transportation on land - Transportation by air - Car rentals - Cruises - Organized tours - Health insurance - Medical note - Inadequacies - Riots in destination countries - Medical equipment - Documenting the matter - Office - Transportation of medications and syringes in air - Camping in the woods - Unexpected traffic jam - Planes, trains, or buses may be delayed - Not packed in time - Don't get enough sleep - Arrange to get both kids a little snack - Forget to bring extra Epi-Pen - Don't forget the 'dog' bag.

To provide swimming lessons over spring break, July, and August, the parent of a daycare child with multiple food allergies often drove an hour and 30 minutes each way. The trepidation of the children that they may be allergic to something is well known to her. A parent must think of every possible negative scenario and emotionally prepare himself or herself for the adventure when traveling far and wide on vacation with a child who has multiple food allergies. He or she must also make plans to avoid unpleasant circumstances as best as possible. We find comfort in the knowledge that a parent should know how to make everything as secure as possible after considering every conceivable disaster or catastrophe. The planning phase should be as relaxing as the vacation itself. In this same spirit, we offer the following guidance and considerations to help ensure a successful vacation for the whole family when traveling with an allergic child.

Aspects to travel: Preparatory steps

10. Celebrating Holidays and Special Occasions

Jessica wants her wedding to be the first truly joyous occasion we've celebrated. We started clinging to some Jewish holy days and Sabbath observances after Ella was diagnosed with food allergies. We had not been observant of them before, and we are very casual about our observance. But, the traditions we have incorporated are the ones that I think could make life more pleasant and, to an extent, less stuffed. There are no specific foods that Jennie cannot eat at Passover, if you can get your hands on the supervised-for-Passover egg substitute. But, there are many foods that we stay away from. We take the opportunity every year at our small seder to remember how unpleasant dishes have made us, and that bread passes over nothing more than our daughter's esophagus. Of course, my attitude is very different, but shared: "You told Mommy a big, big bit pretty bird, and pretty [other host of the event], pretty Duck [Jennie]. Maine!"

It hasn't been easy watching others around us celebrate holidays and special occasions with no awareness of the profound changes that our family has had to make to do the same. I wasn't initially thrilled that our retreat to the Outer Banks took place over Thanksgiving weekend last year. It meant that Ella was left out of her school's Thanksgiving Day "feast", featuring historically accurate foods. And, because we couldn't shop for my side of the family holiday and plan and prepare Ella-safe foods,

Thanksgiving was not very festive. I made a small turkey breast, but we had neither fresh nor dried sage for the dressing. We didn't have or make time for cranberry sauce; it wasn't Ella-safe, and she wouldn't eat it anyway. I hadn't made a pumpkin pie in many years and had to track down last year's can to verify it was dairy- and egg-free. Thomas the Turkey, a buttery shortbread edible-nest-housed turkey at the head of this blog, is hanging out to let you know that he wasn't eaten.

Public or private organizations are showing awareness in considering the experiences of adults and family members living with a variety of dietary restrictions by creating levels of inclusive dining. It is equally, if not more, important to host inclusive celebrations and build slightly more involved logistics of inclusive activities and food options. Including children with food restrictions shows that the welfare of a child is paramount; the basis for which many organizations were created. Often, children are forgotten in these events because they are children and "don't have a voice." Imparting the best opportunity for a child to feel not "left out" of these events has spillover effects on self-esteem and overall positive mental health.

Schools and other community organizations often host special events or occasions that take the form of a birthday party, luncheon, or celebration. To include all children, regardless of their dietary allergen restrictions, requires advance planning on the part of the parent and persuasion on the part of the school or organization to have allergen-free food options. Nuts are often a universal allergen. Check in with the parent first to see if they will allow the child to eat a slice of cake or pizza. Be open and tout the idea of "inclusion" - the intent to help this idea "scale up" in the school, district, and community for inclusion in as many school-based events as possible.

11. Research and Innovation in Allergy Management

Physicians at Mount Sinai Hospital in New York are currently working to improve egg oral immunotherapy using baked egg goods for children with egg allergy. In Hoffmann's ongoing protocols, they are able to enroll children with multiple food allergies or other significant health issues, making interpretation of food allergy trial data less generalizable to the food allergy population as a whole.

Many research studies are focused on the identification of factors indicating which children may be more likely to have severe or persistent food allergies. Some emerging topics in the realm of food allergies include studies investigating the impact of environmental influences on food allergies. Multiple studies are monitoring how the newer treatments being tested might be making a difference, but since none of these treatments are approved for both egg and milk allergies, results may not be generalizable.

As anaphylactic events have decreased in the general population, research must instead rely on patient self-reporting or accidental exposure studies. Accidental allergen ingestion is common among children with a milk and an egg allergy, and one of the main reasons why tolerance studies are difficult to enroll.

As time progressed, we saw the landscape of food allergy management evolve. We observed emerging treatments for multiple allergen families, including monotherapy and in some instances dual therapy, offering great strides for individuals with peanut allergies. These therapies are currently in clinical trial phases for the treatment of additional allergens, some with and without dual therapy options. A phase 2 clinical trial investigating a drug that could be used to treat FPIES reactions is also underway. Quickly disintegrating tablets, patches, and other products that could simplify epinephrine administration during a reaction are also currently in various stages of acquisition. These current treatments, as well as those currently being studied, hold promise for the future of food allergy management.

11.1. Emerging Treatments

The management of food allergies is about to go through much advancement. The path forward will likely involve prevention of allergies or the treatment of existing allergies with several allergens in the long term. This could imply being able to eat a wide variety of foods one day for Layla. There are even trials ongoing now that involve creating allergy "vaccines" for multiple allergies. For large allergies, studies are already showing some success and a reduction in allergen-reactive cells and importance of quality of care on outcomes. In a study from AllerGen, receiving good chronic disease management that met individual patient needs as well as care by a pediatrician were associated with higher quality of life scores in children with food allergy.

Immunotherapies such as the commercialized Palforzia oral immunotherapy (OIT) and the nascent Viaskin peanut patch and AR101 (Layla and Layla + AR201) therapies for peanut allergies have been well studied. There are also other modalities, such as oral mucus antibody treatments, on the horizon. OIT is reliant on the intake of controlled doses of the allergen, whereas the Viaskin patch uses epicutaneous (skin) administration, making it more accessible to be administered and reducing the risk of anaphylactic reactions. Meanwhile, most allergic reactions to cow's milk do not decrease over time and there is no treatment for multiple food allergies.

12. Conclusion

A diagnosis of multiple food allergies in children, while challenging and debilitating for families, provides an opportunity for people to understand the importance of an inclusive society and recognize the resilience of families when faced with significant challenges in the 21st century. This essay delves into the world of parents and how they journey alongside their child with multiple food allergies as they grow up to become confident and empathetic adults. Much of the focus has been on managing the risks of severe allergic reactions in food-allergic children and the impact on their psychological and emotional well-being. Changing family and community cultures can be bittersweet, full of challenges and triumphs, as captured in the story that follows.

In conclusion, having a child with multiple food allergies is challenging, frustrating, and sometimes heart-wrenching. Yet, being a part of a small community of parents who can relate to your struggles and triumphs is truly a beautiful thing. The path of life is never smooth and the journey is seemingly never-ending. I have chosen positive thinking and a glass half full mentality to help navigate the challenges. Although I am unsure of the cause of my son's eczema, embracing the various treatments as a proactive measure is something that I can control, lowering my sense of guilt knowing full well that I have tried to help clear the path for my son from the beginning.

12.1. Reflections on the Journey

EPILOGUE: The journey took so long - fourteen-plus years - that I lost track of time. Looking back, ours has been a life of struggle, triumph, pain, frustration, success, sorrow, joy, regression, laughter, fear, friendship, and above all, love. We all have increased our pain tolerance and grown with the trials, tribulations, transitions, and love involved since before, and especially after the arrival of Brian Christopher. Hazel and I know we and our other kids are better people because we were the parents to Brian. We helped to polish a special, unique gem. In spite of the fact that our smiles have been wiped away now for a while, we wouldn't trade the time we had. We cherish its memory, but we could never go back now. All we ever wanted was for our beautiful son to be healthy and happy so he could realize his dreams. After all is said and done, Brian owns the most important things on earth: the unbroken spirit of love, family, friendships, and the knowledge that he has both eternally steadfast and loving parents.

For the past several weeks, I've been sharing excerpts from the book I wrote about the journey, many detours and some triumphs, of my son Brian's fourteen-year journey through life with Hazel, my wife and his mother. This week I'm providing an excerpt I wrote as the epilogue to the book, something I consider to be the most important thing I've ever written. I wanted to wrap up leaving no questions about how our family felt after such an arduous journey together.

FX: The Hardest Part of the Journey wrap-up music.